Chemo and Me
My Hair Loss Experience

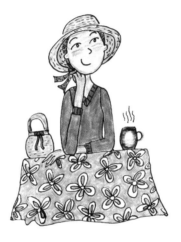

Written and Illustrated by
Tani Miller

Published by the American Cancer Society
Health Promotions
250 Williams Street NW
Atlanta, Georgia 30303 USA

Printed in Mexico
5 4 3 2 1   09 10 11 12 13

For more information about cancer, contact your American Cancer Society at
1-800-ACS-2345 or www.cancer.org.

For bulk sales, please e-mail the American Cancer Society at
trade.sales@cancer.org.

Library of Congress Cataloging-in-Publication Data
Miller, Tāni.
   Chemo and me: my hair loss experience/written and illustrated by Tāni Miller.
       p. cm.
   ISBN-13: 978-1-60443-009-7 (hardcover: alk. paper)
   ISBN-10: 1-60443-009-5 (hardcover: alk. paper)
   1. Miller, Tāni—Health. 2. Cancer—Patients—United States—Biography.
   3. Cancer—Chemotherapy—Complications. 4. Baldness. 5. Cancer in women.
   I. Title.

   RC265.6.M55A3 2009
   616.99'40610092—dc22
   [B]

2008048564

AMERICAN CANCER SOCIETY
Strategic Director, Content: Chuck Westbrook
Director, Cancer Information: Terri Ades, MS, FNP-BC, AOCN
Director, Book Publishing: Len Boswell
Book Marketing/Rights Manager: Candace Magee
Managing Editor, Books: Rebecca Teaff, MA
Books Editor: Jill Russell
Book Publishing Coordinator: Vanika Jordan, MSPub
Editorial Assistant, Books: Amy Rovere

This book is dedicated to—

God, my rock and my provider.

Sue Whitehouse, who climbs mountains and
inspires me to greater heights of my own.
Your friendship opens my mind, fills me with
laughter, and gives me confidence
to face new challenges.

All the wonderful, fun, supportive girls
I work with at Treasure Cove.

Prior to chemotherapy and with the help of my hairdresser, I went out and bought a very nice wig that closely matched my hair color and style.

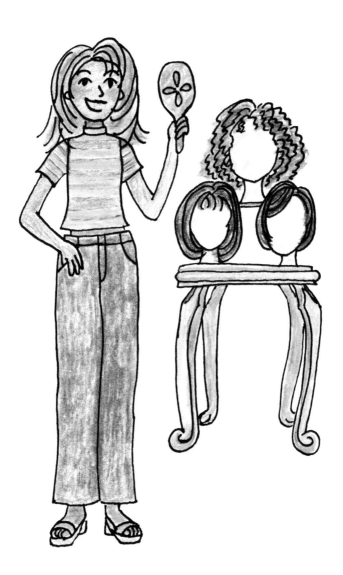

I also bought many hats, scarves, and bandanas. Experimenting with those headcoverings before losing my hair gave me a sense of security and preparedness.

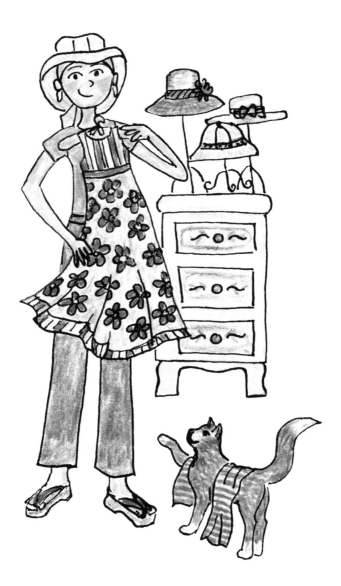

But all of my planning did not work out. For instance, when my hair began to fall out, my head became very sore to the touch. So some of the hats hurt, and some were now too big.

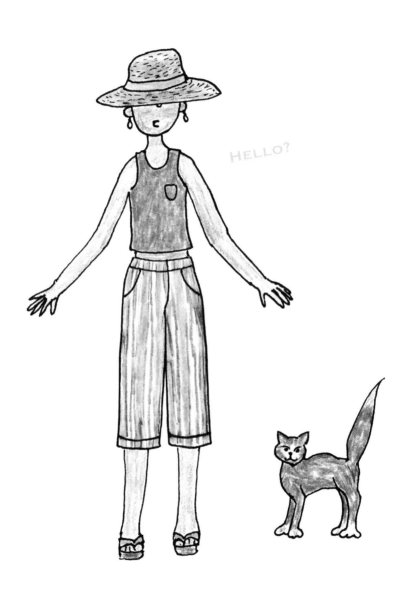

Although I had bought a wig, it never felt quite right for me and I never once wore it. However, many of the other wigs that were given to me were perfect for freaking out my friends!

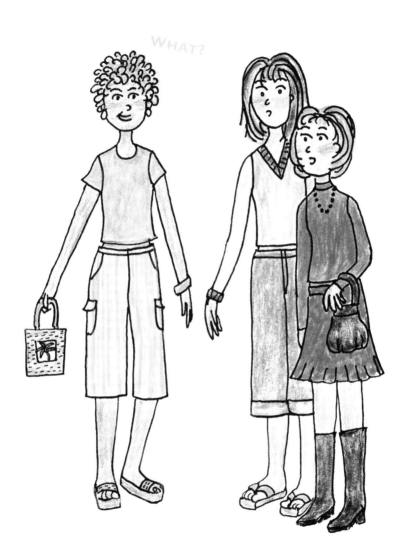

The hat that became my favorite was made of soft white terry cloth. Luckily, I had bought several just like it. It felt soft and comforting on my sore head, and the snug fit kept it secure in the wind. I wore this type of hat with brightly colored bandanas. The look was sporty—perfect for my casual style.

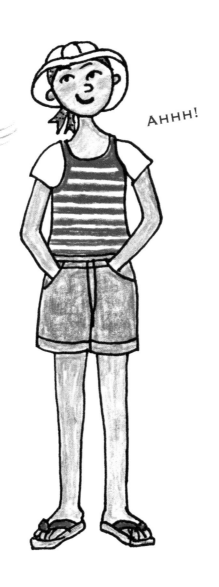

AHHH!

My best discovery was to frequently use a sticky lint roller to clear my head of continually loosening hair. That way, it did not end up on my shoulders or elsewhere in my surroundings.

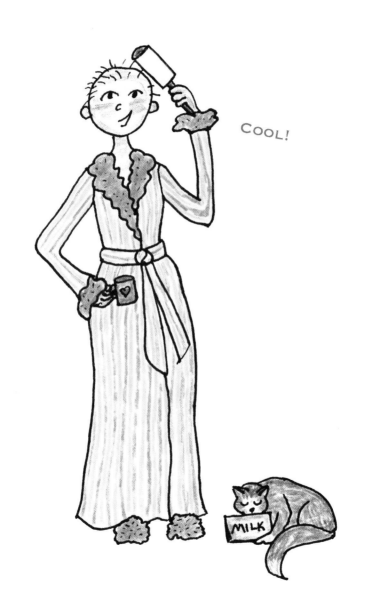

COOL!

MILK

There were some positive things that came with hair loss. I saved a small fortune in haircuts, colorings, and hair products.

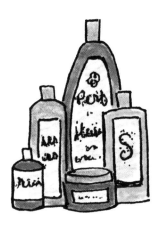

The bathroom floor stayed
hair free.

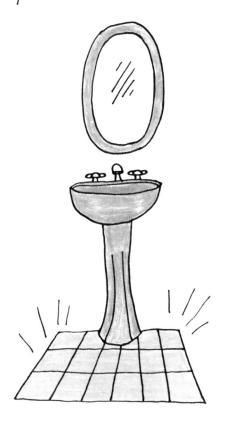

Because I no longer had to spend time styling my hair, I slept in an extra half hour every day.

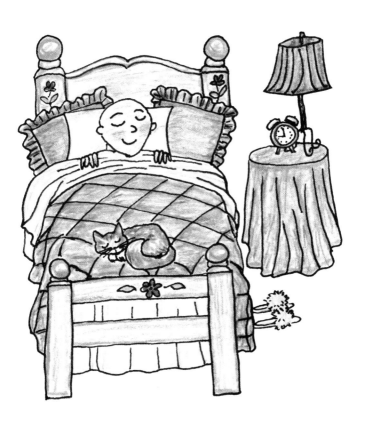

However, some things were very aggravating. While applying mascara, my eyelashes came off on the brush.

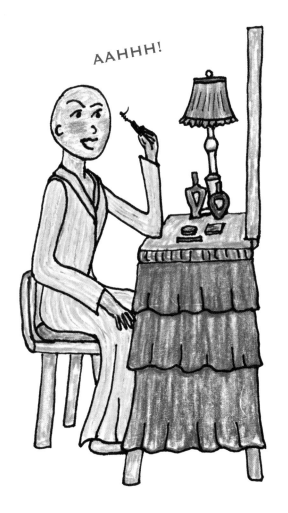

I still grew hair where I did not want it, and I still had to shave my legs.

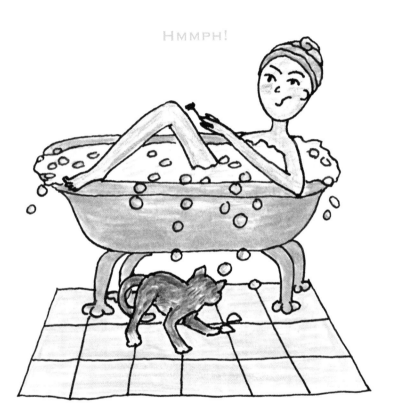

Then one day it all got to be too much. I didn't feel well, and when I looked in the mirror I didn't even recognize myself.

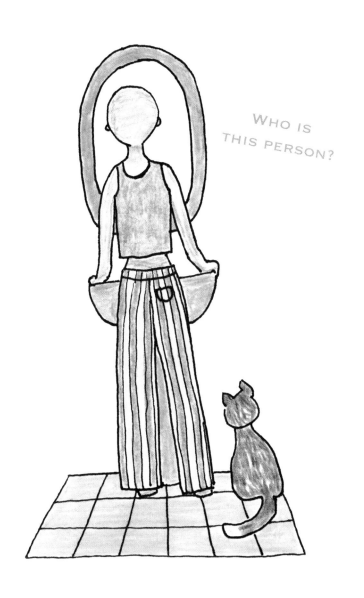

WHO IS
THIS PERSON?

I figured the only way I could improve my looks at that point was to smile. So that's what I did. I started to smile. I started to smile a lot!

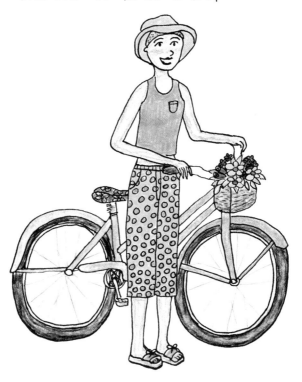

Then I noticed people were smiling back, and before I knew it I felt happy.

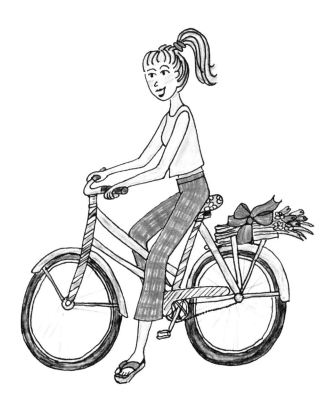

I guess a part of me thought people were going to reject me when I lost my hair, but instead I found them to be incredibly kind. I began to see my illness as having a purpose. It wasn't completely about me. It gave others a chance to shine and feel good about themselves. And it made it okay for me to relax and accept their gifts of love. I began to feel free just to be me! This led to new hobbies...

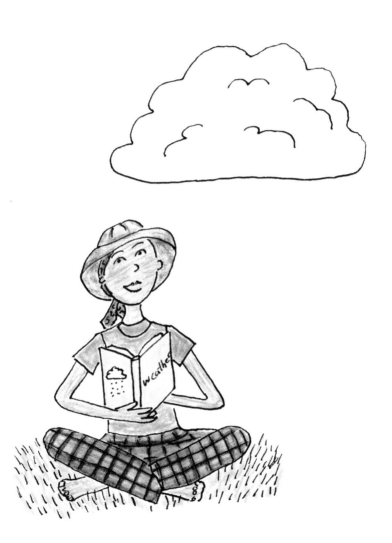

Revival of old ones...

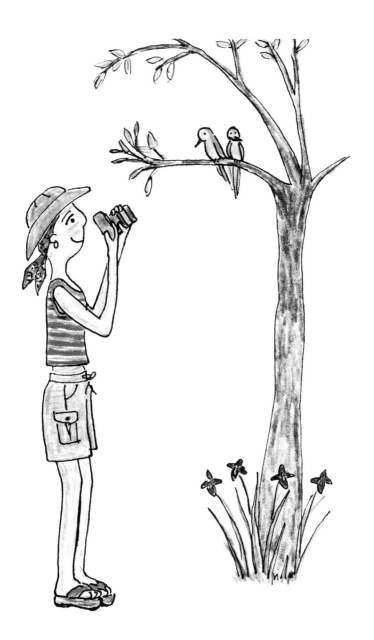

And aspirations for new!

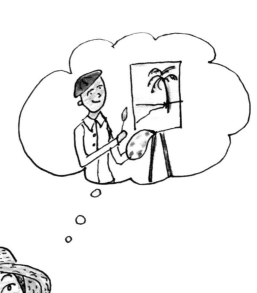
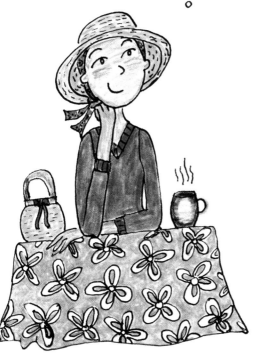

Then, just as I began to enjoy all the newfound freedoms, I looked in the mirror and I had sprouts! At first it was just a five o'clock shadow. But soon...

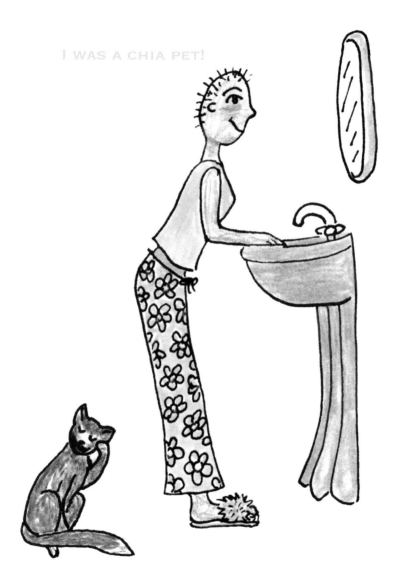

I can say most people never noticed I had lost my hair. In fact, my hat and scarf ensembles actually brought me more compliments. So I can tell you, if you do lose your hair...

Some people will think you look hip!

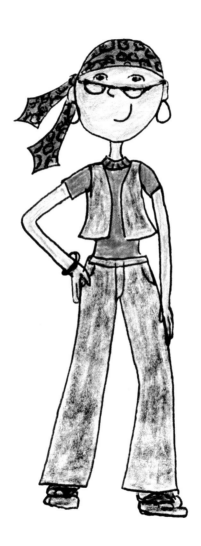

Some people will think you look sporty!

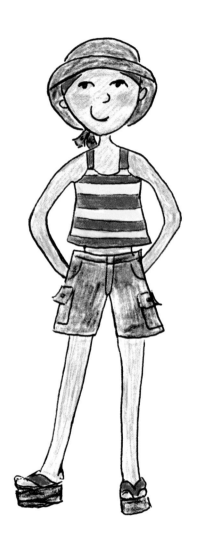

Some people will think you look chic!

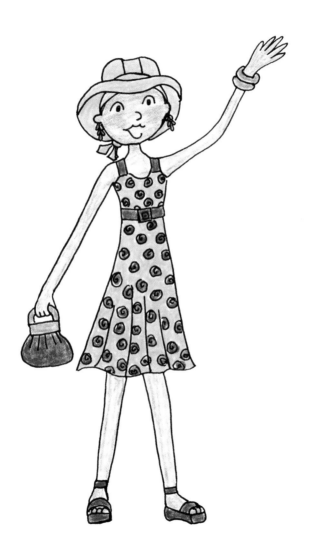

But most of all, the people who know you and love you will think how incredibly brave you are!

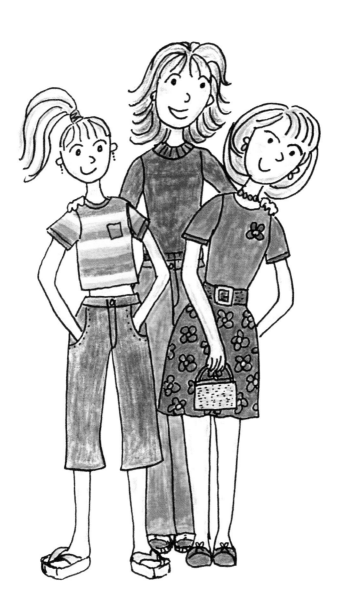

Oh! And if you pull your bandana really tight, it gives you an instant eyelift!

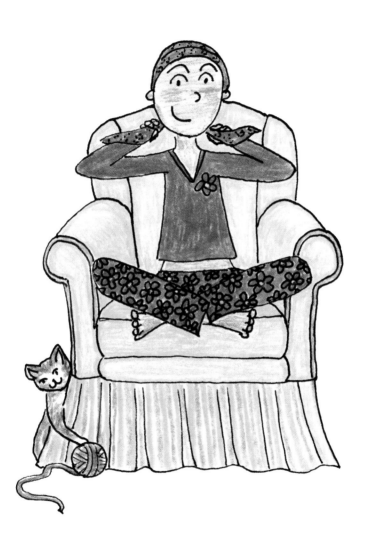

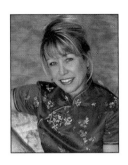

Tani Miller resides in Ormond Beach, Florida, where she operates her store, Treasure Cove Consignments. After an eye-opening breast cancer diagnosis in 2004, she began writing and illustrating. She also combined her love of nature, wildlife, and photography into a successful line of photographic greeting cards and prints.